I0442055

Secrets of a Happy Healthy Working Girl

Secrets of a Happy Healthy Working Girl

A Small Change Approach to Wellness at Work

Kimberly Petrosino

Copyright © 2016 Kimberly Petrosino
All rights reserved.

ISBN-13: 9781530285082
ISBN-10: 1530285089

Disclaimer

THE CONTENTS OF this book is for informational purposes only. It is not intended to prevent, diagnose or treat any illnesses and is not meant to replace the reader's relationship with their physician or other medical professional or healthcare practitioner. Please consult your doctor for specific matters pertaining to your health and diet.

Dedication

To Mom and Joanne, for being the only sure thing in my life when everything else was changing. None of this would be possible if it weren't for your support and your unconditional love. I may not always say much but my gratitude runs deep. No matter what ups and downs I face, I never lose sight of everything you've done for me. You are the single two most important people in the world to me.

"I don't think any other animal knows the difference between Monday and Tuesday"

— DEEPAK CHOPRA

Table of Contents

Introduction

"Bottom line: You only live once. Let's keep the stress to a minimum."

— Kimberly Petrosino, *The Small Change Solution*

When I was a 20 year old college student, I was met with a proposition from my then-boss: "You can have a promotion, if you work full time." I should have been making friends, doing homework, joining clubs and enjoying college life. Instead, I took the promotion and from then on I ran back and forth between school and work every day, for no reason other than I was a people-pleaser and a go-getter. It wasn't because I needed the money. I lived at home and my parents provided for me (although I was financing a rather lofty shopping habit).

I would never say I regretted the choice I made back then; regret is a really strong word and if I had turned down the promotion and got the quintessential college experience, my life would have turned out totally different. I simply wouldn't recommend it to anyone in that position. I have no college friends, no college memories. I never attended a football game, a school play, or a party. I didn't have a favorite teacher, I didn't spend the week before finals holed up with everyone else in the library. I don't even really remember anyone's name. I took as many online classes as I could so that I had more availability to give my job.

I'm sure this sounds familiar to a lot of you, especially those of you who didn't have a choice but to work through college - which let's face it, these days, is most of us. But it sure is sad looking back ten years later and realizing you don't have a single fond memory from what is supposed to be the "greatest four years of your life". (Which on an unrelated note, I totally disagree with. Early thirties is where it's at. Until I'm in my late thirties, then those will be the greatest years. And so on. You get the idea.)

I tried for a do-over by going to grad school, but I was still working full time so it was the same story again. All I could say is that time I made studying more of a priority and I came through with a far more impressive GPA.

That was more than a decade ago. Since then, the company I worked for remained the only constant in my otherwise tumultuous twenties. The various stages of my life brought with it varying stages of health. My weight went up and down and back up again. I went through periods of getting Chinese take-out every day, thinking if I walked down the block to pick it up instead of driving then the food wouldn't count against me. I would go through a bag of baked chips every time I had to work a double shift – but that's fine, because they're baked, right? I didn't know a thing about nutrition. Even the year I started dabbling in vegetarianism, it was all about the PB&J's and heavy pasta.

My journey to better health has been a slow, upward climb. After years on the roller coaster of weight loss and gain and emotional instability, which I now know to be the result of poor diet choices, I finally feel in balance (most days, anyway) and eager to share my secrets with you.

I take a "small change" approach to life, never overwhelming myself with more changes than I can adjust to easily. I don't do anything "cold turkey". The reason for this is that generally when people make a drastic change to their lifestyle, like waking up one morning and deciding they are no longer a coffee drinker, it tends not to stick. When reading this book, I don't recommend you try to implement every suggestion all at once. Incorporate them naturally into your everyday life as you feel comfortable.

Working Girl's Exercise

Set an intention. What is it that you want to get out of this book? Better time management skills? To learn how to better separate home and work life? Think of 2-3 intentions and write them down.

_____

_____

_____

What action steps will you take to help you achieve this?

_____

_____

_____

CHAPTER 1

Good Morning, Sunshine!

YOUR FIRST STEPS in the morning set the entire day in motion. That's not to say that if you spend an hour journaling, meditating, and doing yoga in the morning, your entire day will be serene and peaceful. Unfortunately that lies at the mercy of the nature of your job. Likewise, if you have a chaotic morning, it doesn't necessarily mean that your entire day will be equally insane. I believe that how you approach the first hour or two of your day stimulates you in a way that will affect how you handle anything the rest of the day brings.

Case in point: My mornings can go either one of three ways – I can get up early for a workout before starting my day (rare, but it has happened), I can get up 60-90 minutes prior to leaving for the office for some productive quiet time, or I can get up 30 minutes before leaving for the office and run around like a stressed-out nut praying I haven't forgotten anything. Those three scenarios give me **VERY** different results for how I carry myself the rest of the day. If I can get in an AM workout, I can tackle the day super energetic and ready for anything. If I have an hour or so to myself in the morning to quietly but fully prepare myself for the day ahead, then I feel calm and collected all day. If I oversleep and race out the door in less time than it takes to double check that my hair is brushed, all bets are off. I get tired and irritable and my coffee intake goes up considerably. I suspect that if I started every day that way, in the long run my health would suffer.

Take a moment to imagine how you would ideally approach each day, if you had the choice. Guess what – you DO have the choice! You've heard the phrase "fake it 'til you make it". Act like a morning person, and eventually you'll become one.

That being said, make sure your morning routine reflects you. I encourage you to be open minded and try out different things, but if you're genuinely not a morning gym-goer, don't force yourself to become one. I couldn't do it. I loved the feeling of having an abundant amount of energy AND knowing that my workout was already done, but on a daily basis it's too much for me first thing in the morning (especially during the dark winter months). Other people thrive on AM workouts. Figure out what makes you feel balanced and centered in the morning, and do it every day. When you begin to feel stressed out during the day, harness that positive energy. And if you do occasionally oversleep and leave the house with two different shoes on, take a deep breath and begin again. You have the power to start your day over at any time.

Working Girl's Exercise

What does your ideal morning look like? Do you have time to read the newspaper, maybe take a walk? Write down, in detail, your perfect morning.

_____

_____

_____

What action steps will you take to create your perfect morning? (Ex. "I will wake up five minutes earlier" or "I will prepare my lunch the night before")

_____

_____

_____

CHAPTER 2

Embracing Your Daily Commute

"There will always be rocks in the road ahead of us. They will be stumbling blocks or stepping stones, it all depends on how you use them."

— FRIEDRICH NIETZSCHE

To you, the daily commute might mean an hour stuck in gridlock amongst a sea of other angry, sleep-deprived travelers. To me, it is an hour of sanctuary before a busy day. An hour to catch up on my playlist or talk out a problem (and hope the driver of the adjacent car isn't looking at me).

The typical nine-to-fiver spends enough time in the car or on public transportation that how you handle it can have an effect on your health. Several years ago, I was offered a job that was better in nature and in salary but meant a longer commute. As someone who is easily offended by the antics of other people on the road (like the guy in the big truck *really* cut me off because he hated me personally), I took control of the situation from the start. I ordered a book on tape and a CD to help me re-learn Italian. I loaded up my iPod and my supply of road trip snacks and I was ready for anything! (Just so we're clear though, I still can't speak more than ten words of Italian.)

Here are a few other ways to keep your commute stress-free and healthy:

Watch your posture. This is something VERY few people are conscious of, but it's so important. Sit up straight. It will take some focus at first, but you will get used to it. In this day of everyone walking around while staring at their phones 24/7, I worry that in time we will all be in a permanent state of looking down.

Crack the window. I am OBSESSED with getting fresh air! Even in the winter I try to open the window for a few minutes while I'm driving. It just perks me up. Take in a few deep, cleansing breaths and see how much better you feel.

Stash some basic cleaning supplies somewhere in your car. I'm just saying, if you're not disinfecting your steering wheel regularly, who is?

Keep your cell phone in the backseat. Okay so that's more a safety precaution than a health tip, but it's still worth mentioning.

If your commute is a nightmare, you are starting the day off on the wrong foot. This is one of those things you really have no control over unless you change either your job or your place of residence. An enjoyable ride to the office really doesn't call for such drastic measures (usually). Try to shift your mindset and see if you can turn it into "me" time.

Bonus tip: I once heard a suggestion on the radio that I thought was fantastic. Every time you're stuck in traffic, think of a way you can tell someone in your life "I appreciate you". We often don't have the time to share our gratitude with those who deserve it most, especially as busy professionals. So what better time than while you're not going anywhere fast anyway?

Working Girl's Exercise

How you do feel about your morning commute? Does it make you bored, restless, cranky, or even angry? How do you wish your commute made you feel? What can you change that you DO have control over?

_____

_____

_____

What action steps will you take to help you achieve this? (Ex. "I will set up a 'Happy Morning!' playlist to pump me up during my commute" or "I will leave a few minutes earlier to avoid traffic")

_____

_____

_____

CHAPTER 3

The Friend/Coworker Balance

I USED TO like to keep my personal life separate from life at the office. While others chatted about their weekends and their kids and their doctors' appointments, I usually kept to myself. For one thing, I'm a pretty private person and I know how quickly gossip can spread. I've also seen how quickly drama can spread, especially when you're dealing with one or two "toxic" people. You know who I'm talking about. Every office has one. This is the one who spews negativity and hates everything. They're energy vampires. They despise happy people.

Don't allow yourself to get sucked in. When the conversation gets heated, politely excuse yourself by saying you need to get back to work. If someone tries to get you to take sides in an argument, simply say you don't want to get involved. There's no way to 100% avoid office drama. You spend more time with your coworkers than you do your families, and every now and then you're bound to bump heads with someone. But if you can stay out of it for the most part and remain neutral on any issues that arise among the people surrounding you, you will have a lot less anxiety to deal with.

With that being said, it can be a little lonely if you don't have at least one or two close coworkers – someone you can vent to on occasion, or share good news with. Perhaps you're lucky enough to have a group of work friends you like to get together with outside of the office once in a while.

Not everyone thrives in an office setting. Let's face it, it's unnatural. Maybe you're someone who works better alone, or maybe you prefer to keep to yourself. Maybe you have been placed near people you just can't stand. But the fact remains that you're in it, and if you can't change your situation, you *can* change the way you react to it.

Working Girl's Exercise

How well do you interact with others at work? Do you prefer to keep to yourself, or do you excel in group situations? Everyone is different. Where would you like to be in this area?

_____

_____

_____

What action steps will you take to help you achieve this?

_____

_____

_____

CHAPTER 4

The Art of Healthy Snacking

I'M JUST GOING to jump right in with rule #1: Avoid vending machines at all costs. Even the "healthy" stuff – you can do so much better than that, just as easily, and best of all, cheaper! I have an airtight glass jar in my kitchen with the words "Trail Mix" written on the chalkboard label. I don't know if its contents are really considered trail mix; maybe more like "Random Mix". Every other week or so when I'm running low I'll pick up nuts – almonds, walnuts, pistachios, pecans – and something sweet, like raisins, dates or dried cranberries. Whatever it is goes right into the jar so it's never the same mix, but whatever it is, it's power-packed and healthy. I either eat it as is, or mix it with rolled oats, organic peanut butter and a little raw honey for a quick and easy homemade energy bar.

I usually snack twice a day – mid-morning and mid-afternoon. In the morning, veggie sticks and hummus is the perfect pick-me-up. Store bought hummus is fine, just buy organic if possible so you can avoid any artificial colors, flavors, or chemicals that are found in certain brands. In the afternoon (sometimes known as the mid-afternoon slump, when people are usually reaching for a second cup of coffee – we will dive deeper into this in Chapter Twelve!), I'll either grab a handful of my home-made Random Mix or a piece of dark chocolate (at least 70% cacao).

A good rule of thumb is to eat every two to three hours, and let no more than five hours go by without eating something. This means that over the course of a standard workday, you're looking at lunch and two snacks. Of course you should do what feels right for you, but a daily meal plan of mine might look a little like this:

7am – Breakfast of a green smoothie and organic oatmeal

10-11am – Snack of hummus and veggie sticks

2pm – Lunch of quinoa on a wrap with avocado on top and a creamy vegetable soup on the side

4pm – Afternoon snack of dark chocolate or trail mix

7pm – Dinner of quinoa and steamed vegetables

After dinner, if I feel like I need a little something, I'll snack on ginger snaps or organic popcorn with my hot tea. For the most part though, I stop eating three to four hours before I go to bed.

Everyone is different, but I find that eating several small meals a day is ideal. Each meal or snack gives me the energy I need to power through the next few hours, and all of my energy is not being used to digest food.

In Chapter Nine we will get into a few nutritional basics for the workplace, but when it comes to snacking keep these things in mind: avoid artificial colors, flavors and chemicals, make sure you can pronounce all of the ingredients, and snack on whole foods whenever possible (bonus points if it's organic!).

Working Girl's Exercise

When you're craving something during the workday, what do you tend to gravitate towards? A bag of chips, maybe some chocolate?

_____

_____

_____

Start small, resolve to add in one "clean" snack a day. List three healthy snacks you can incorporate into your day for a non-caffeine-induced boost.

_____

_____

_____

CHAPTER 5

Get Moving

"Nothing will work unless you do."

— Maya Angelou

THE AVERAGE CUBICLE inhabitant sits for the majority of the day. There are *countless* studies out there reporting that sitting down all day can negatively impact your health over time. Working out at the beginning or end of each day won't counteract the effects, either. You have to find ways to move your body throughout the day to lessen the impact of sitting on your health.

Here are a few simple suggestions to incorporate more movement into your daily routine:

Stand whenever possible. If you work at a computer of course you need to sit while you're typing, but can you stand to flip through your files or make phone calls? You may feel a little awkward at first but it's unlikely anyone around you will even notice.

If you can't stand while you work, move around for a few minutes every hour. Walk to the copier, the water cooler, the restroom, or go chat with a coworker for a few minutes. If you can't leave your desk, at least take a few minutes to stretch. Roll your shoulders, shake out your wrists and ankles, and do some side twists.

Park further away and take the stairs. These are two of the most commonly suggested ways to add steps into your day but hey, it's with good reason! If you can't take the stairs all the way to your floor, walk one or two flights and get on the elevator from there. As you get comfortable, add in a few more. When you need to use the restroom, use one on a different floor and take the stairs to get there. If you need to talk to a coworker on another floor, walk over instead of calling.

Eat before you sign out for lunch (if you can) and use your lunch break to walk instead. If you're not allowed to eat at your desk, arrive at work a few minutes early or leave a few minutes later and walk then. At least that way you'll avoid traffic! I always find that a light walk after a meal helps me to digest it, so if possible try to walk for at least a few minutes after eating lunch rather than sitting right back down at your desk.

Team up! Find someone else in your office who likes to walk and take your lunch break together. Having someone to chat with will make it more fun!

No one ever woke up one morning after a lifelong sedentary existence and ran a marathon (I'm guessing). It takes time. You have to get your sneakers on. Get comfortable running for five minutes. Then ten. Then an hour. And so on. Just because you can't do it now doesn't mean you can't do it *ever.*

Allow me to share a personal story. Just a few short years ago I was overweight and out of shape. The last time I had run was in high school, and that was because I *had* to. I was depressed and feeling badly about myself during what should have been a very exciting time in my life. At 27 years old, I was living on my own for the first time and getting my first taste of independence. I could do what I wanted, *when* I wanted. But all I could think was, I feel terrible. I LOOK terrible. This isn't the life I want.

One night in the middle of winter I felt a surge of empowerment: *I'm going to go for a run.* Just a short one, around the field and back. A total distance of maybe half a mile.

I dusted off my old sneakers – and I'm talking OLD, I wasn't even sure I had sneakers prior to that night – went outside, and starting jogging. By the time I reached the end of my block, four houses away, I felt as though my lungs would explode. I could barely breathe. I was crushed, and very nearly accepted defeat that night. I didn't factor in that running in twenty degree weather when you have no experience is the worst thing you can do. All I knew is I'd failed.

Soon after that night, I read about a popular new app that provided users with a running plan, a journal, a timer, and encouragement. I downloaded it immediately and put my sneakers on once more. For the next nine weeks, I went outside and ran. I started at thirty seconds on, thirty seconds off, and slowly worked my way up. Soon I was running for five minutes without stopping, then twenty, then thirty. I set goals for myself and when I reached one, I set another. One mile, then two. My first 5k. My first 5k without stopping to walk. Then 10k. Then, two and a half years later, my first half marathon. As I write this, I'm training for my third half marathon.

I now know that night to be an enormous turning point in my life. If I had given up and continued to live my life that way, I wouldn't have anything I have now. I wouldn't have gone on to become a Health Coach. I wouldn't have written my first book, "The Small Change Solution", and I wouldn't have written this one. I wouldn't have connected with hundreds of amazing people on my path to a healthier lifestyle (including you!). I certainly wouldn't be running half marathons – basically, I would have settled into a life I *thought* I was living fully without ever really knowing what I was capable of. Truth be told, I STILL don't know what I'm capable of. A little bit more is revealed to me with every passing day.

We have to lose the "all or nothing" mentality when it comes to moving our bodies and getting exercise. You may not have time to put in an hour at the gym, but you certainly have time to take a ten minute walk every night (yes, you do. No excuses.). Start thinking of it as MAKING time, not HAVING time. Sure you're busy, but you don't HAVE to do everything you're doing, you CHOOSE to. That hour every week you spend at the nail salon? You could be taking a yoga class. I'm not saying you *should*, I'm just trying to shift your perspective. You HAVE the time, it's a matter of how you USE the time. We all get the same 24 hours in a day! If you can't/won't go to the gym, you can still make huge strides in your health by finding easy ways to move your body throughout the day. Small changes add up, and they inspire other small changes. Over time, you will see BIG results. Stick with it – and if all you have is five minutes, blast your favorite power song and dance it out!

Food for thought: Look ahead three years. Where do you wish you could be? What do you wish you could do? What can you do *right now*?

What is YOUR "running story"? Write it down, and figure out how to make it happen.

Working Girl's Exercise

When it comes to physical activity, how are you doing? Are you a regular gym goer? Do you wish you could find more ways to add movement into your day? What does your ideal day look like in terms of exercise?

_____

_____

_____

Remember, it's all about the small changes. What action steps will you take to help you achieve your physical activity goals? (Ex. "I will take the stairs" or "I will arrive at work 20 minutes earlier to walk before my shift")

_____

_____

_____

CHAPTER 6

Curing the Monday Blues

"You don't need a new year to make a fresh start. All you need is a Monday."

— UNKNOWN

IF YOU'VE EVER seen the movie *Office Space*, you know "Sounds like someone's got a case of the Mondays", and you know it well. Mondays are wildly unpopular in our society, and I think it's time we all change our way of thinking and start embracing the first day of the new week with as warm a welcome as we give the first day of a new year.

How do we do this, you ask? Here are a few suggestions to get you started:

Prepare in advance. One of life's biggest bummers (in my opinion) is spending more time at work/preparing for work/thinking about work than you do anything else. What can you do on Sunday night to help you get ready for the week? Lay out a few outfits, complete with accessories. Make sure the car is gassed and ready to go, and you're armed with a fresh playlist for the commute. Prepare a lunch that will have you WISHING it was Monday already!

Think of it as a fresh start. You say first day of a *long* week, I say first day of a BRAND NEW week! It's all about the mindset. You wanted a fresh start? It's here. The first thing I do on Monday mornings is take out a snazzy piece of stationary, date it with the week at hand, and start writing my goals. I start with the big ones and work my way down to the tiniest detail. I set a few intentions for the week, and finish my "Note to Self" with a quote I'm loving in that moment. Having everything all in one space makes it easy to refer back to throughout the week, and crossing things off as I go is so gratifying! Don't forget: If you're listing some seriously big aspirations (as you should be, you little dreamer, you!) leave some room underneath to break it down into smaller, more manageable steps. For example, if your goal is to save up for a new car, figure out how much you need to set aside on a weekly basis and how many overtime hours you want to work this week to help reach your savings goal. If you simply write "I want to buy a car", you won't know where to start to help you get there. The clearer your goal and the more specific your action steps, the more likely you are to get there.

Plan something mid-week. Every day of the week has a purpose, and for Wednesday, that purpose is to grab your girls – or your dudes – have some fun, and forget about work! Having a regularly scheduled mid-week reprieve will give you something to look forward to for the first half of the week, and something to smile about for the second half.

Know who's on your A-Team. Some of your friends are just an email away during the work day – others aren't. Know who you can reach out to during the mid-afternoon slump for a quick laugh or vent session. Sometimes, all you need is a reminder that there is life outside those cubicle walls!

Working Girl's Exercise

New week: Love it or hate it? Remember, sometimes a simple mindset shift is all you need to turn Monday into Mon-YAY! When the first day of the week rolls around, are you coffee-mug-half-empty or coffee-mug-half-full?

_____

_____

_____

What are three things you can do to turn your Monday frown upside-down?

_____

_____

_____

CHAPTER 7

Take Your Break

"There are only so many withdrawals you can make from your health bank account, but you just keep on withdrawing. You could go bankrupt if you don't make some deposits soon."

— ARIANNA HUFFINGTON, *THRIVE*

ACCORDING TO THE Huffington Post, an incredible 42% of Americans took NO vacation time in the year 2014!

WHAT?!

Further research shows that Americans, as a whole, take fewer vacation days a year than in many other countries worldwide.

Be honest, where are you on the time-off spectrum? Do you use every personal day you're allotted, as few as possible, or somewhere in between? What about lunch breaks? Do you eat at your desk and never see the light of day? How about when the clock strikes five – do you go home, or stay at the office burning the midnight oil? Do you answer calls from your boss/clients during non-work hours?

Your answers to these questions can reveal a lot about your health.

Time to get personal again: For a long time, I ate at my desk so I could work through my lunch hour – partially because I was that busy, but also because I enjoyed seeing a few extra dollars in my paycheck every week. Then I got a new manager who didn't allow her staff to skip their breaks, and for that I am forever in her debt.

I still ate at my desk, then I used my free time to take a long walk outside. Once I was away from the office for a few minutes, surrounded by trees and breathing in fresh air, I noticed how much my head cleared. Ideas started flowing through and I instantly felt more relaxed. It wasn't long before I was hooked, and I realized a distinct difference in my mood if I *didn't* take my daily walk.

If you try to power through the whole day without a break, day after day, you're likely to be very tired come 3pm (refer to "Chapter Twelve: Avoid the Mid-Afternoon Slump). Your productivity level will start to diminish based on that alone. If you take a thirty minute break every day, sure, that's a half an hour less you'll spend on that pile of paperwork, but since you'll still be powering on through the mid-afternoon slump, it works out about the same anyway!

It's the same with vacation days. You – mind, body, and spirit – need time to recharge DAILY. If you go years on end without taking a vacation, in the long run it's your health that will suffer. I'm not saying you need to whisk away to an island resort every year (although I certainly encourage it!). A stay-at-home vacation is sometimes all you need to rejuvenate and center yourself.

That said, vacations don't come around that often – so let's talk weekends and non-office hours. How often do you go in on Saturdays? Is your boss constantly calling when you're sitting with your family at the dinner table? You must set clear boundaries when it comes to your working and non-working hours. If the nature of your job requires you to take phone calls or do work from home, you should set office hours – same as you have them from Monday through Friday.

The bottom line is, YES, of course we all need to work to live. Unfortunately, we aren't all blessed with jobs that fulfill our souls. That makes it all the more important to balance out that time with people and activities that *do* fulfill us. If you think that isn't helping you get ahead at the office – trust me, it is. Your more-relaxed, super-productive self is waiting around the corner to tell you so. TAKE. YOUR. BREAKS. End of story.

Okay, fine – if you *really* have to miss your break once in a while (notice I said ONCE IN A WHILE), then make an appointment with yourself for thirty minutes of "me time" immediately after work.

Working Girl's Exercise

Where do you fall on the break scale? Do you take your lunch breaks? Personal days? How about vacations?

_____

_____

_____

What's a reasonable goal for you as far as taking breaks is concerned? (Ex. If you answered "no, never" to the question above, naturally you might not be comfortable immediately scheduling every hour of vacation you're allotted this year.) What action steps will you take to help you achieve this?

_____

_____

_____

CHAPTER 8

Create Your At-Work Oasis

IN MY LAST book, *The Small Change Solution*, I talked about how your home is a reflection of you. If you live in a cluttered space and are constantly searching for things, you are likely to feel a bit scattered and stressed in other areas of your life. On the other hand, if your home is airy and open, full of light and decorated in a manner which soothes your soul, you are likely to move through your day with calm in your heart.

The same applies for the space in which you work. You spend more waking hours at your job than in your home. If your desk is piled high with unorganized papers and day-old coffee cups, if you have dozens of unanswered emails and voicemails, and your office or cubicle itself is overall very dreary… well, that isn't exactly the most welcoming or productive environment.

If management permits it, decorate your desk with plants and pictures of loved ones. Green plants detoxify the air you're breathing (which is especially good considering the limited ventilation in an office building), and photos of loved ones on your desk can bring a smile to your face any time you need one. I also recommend keeping a special word or quote, or preferably several, where you can see them. These notes serve as a reminder to check in, breathe, relax, smile - whatever you need - throughout the day.

Even if your company policy imposes restrictions as to how much personalization you're allowed at your desk, there are still some things you can do. Keep a photograph or other special keepsake in your drawer. Keep your work-space free of clutter. Have clearly marked folders or trays for your "Inbox", "Pending", and "Completed" items. Don't fall behind on your filing system; that will only create chaos. If you're having a particularly busy day, then take five to ten minutes before you go home to get organized. Put all of your papers away, and make a to-do list for tomorrow. Complete whatever you reasonably can before the end of the day or week so it doesn't linger on your mind when you leave the office. Having a routine at the end of your day, rather than making a run for it the moment the hand on the clock reaches that coveted '5', will give you closure so you're not thinking about your unfinished tasks when you should be spending time with your family (or with yourself!).

Working Girl's Exercise

What does your at-work oasis look like? Close your eyes and imagine your dream workspace. Are there plants? Photos? Quotes? Colorful office supplies to brighten up your space? Get specific here!

_____

_____

_____

Working within the parameters of what you're allowed, what steps will you take to create your perfect at-work oasis?

_____

_____

_____

CHAPTER 9

A Crash Course in Nutrition

"Eat food. Not too much. Mostly plants."

— MICHAEL POLLAN

THERE IS A WIDE belief out there that in order to be "healthy", you must be of a certain weight, and to get to that weight, you must count calories, carbs, fat grams, and points. If I even attempted to add up the nutrition facts of everything I ate, all I would think about all day is food! It shouldn't be that hard. I'm about to simplify everything you know about "dieting". (I use quotations because I really hate the notion of diets and all they imply. The word "diet" by definition refers to the kinds of foods a person eats on a regular basis, but the social context of the word of course means something totally different.)

Cook at home more. There's no reason to slave away in the kitchen every single day (unless of course you want to), but make an effort to eat more home cooked meals. Cook with the intention of having leftovers. Portion out those leftovers into smaller containers so you can just grab and go in the morning. Aim to fill those containers halfway with veggies, a quarter healthy whole grains, and a quarter clean protein (and those are guidelines to follow for ALL of your meals).

Plan ahead. Because you cooked with the intention of having leftovers, your meal prep for the next few days is done. Go, you! What else can you do right now to prepare for the week ahead? If I may take the idea of meal prep a step further, I think it's a great idea to wash, chop, and separate your produce as soon as you get it home from the store. Portion out smoothie ingredients into individual bags do you can simply dump the contents into your blender in the morning. Salads can be made in a snap because the veggies are already washed and cut. Before you go grocery shopping, take a few minutes to plan out your meals for the next few days and list the ingredients you need underneath. This might take extra time but it will save you from buying food you don't need, and having a meal plan in place will save you precious moments of standing in front of your refrigerator, surveying its contents and wondering what on earth to make.

Count ingredients, not calories. All calories are not created equal. You might think you're doing good by your diet bringing low-fat freezer meals to work for lunch, right? They seem super convenient because you can stock up on them when they're on sale and just pop one in the microwave for a quick and so-called "healthy" meal. Sure, these meals may contain fewer calories than if you had grabbed lunch from the local drive-thru but what isn't written in big letters on that packaging is that these meals are FULL of sodium and sugar, and who knows what else! They may help you lose weight – at least temporarily – but they are terrible for your health, and that's what's most important here. When choosing packaged food, look carefully at the list of ingredients. If the list is a mile long and full of words you can't pronounce, or if the box says its contents contains artificial colors and flavors, skip it. Strive to eat as many foods as you can that don't HAVE ingredient lists – think fruits, vegetables, and healthy whole grains. Buy organic whenever possible to ensure you're not eating anything artificial.

Live by the rule of 90/10. The rule is simple: Ninety percent of the time, fill your plate (and your glass) with clean, healthy whole foods. The other ten percent of the time, feel free to indulge as you please. You don't have to be totally 90/10 right away. Wherever you feel you fall on that scale, try to increase the ratio a little bit every week. In time, you'll notice that the last ten percent will change completely. My idea of indulgence used to be pizza and Oreo cookies. Now, it's a second cup of coffee in the afternoon.

Always have water. I can't tell you how many weird looks and comments I've gotten in regards to the comically large water bottle I keep with me while I work. If I had a dollar for every time I've said "Yes, I'm finishing the WHOLE THING", I'd be writing this book from a private bungalow in Bora Bora. Drinking water cures plenty of common work-related ailments – like headaches! Try sipping on some before you reach for an aspirin. A commonly suggested rule of thumb is to drink eight to ten glasses of water daily. Truthfully, the ideal amount is different for everyone and is based on many lifestyle factors such as activity level, location, environment and diet. Having a reusable water bottle at your desk, and filling it every morning as soon as you get to the office, makes it much easier to hit your desired water intake. You're going to be there all day anyway, so why not?

Ditch the deprivation theory. Forget about dieting, and forget about "all or nothing". I've already given you the rule of 90/10, and in Chapter Five I told you that just because you may not be able to carve out an hour a day for the gym doesn't mean you can't do *anything*. The same principles apply here. A "cheat moment" does not a "cheat day" make. You can indulge a little without throwing the whole day away. If you want a cupcake, eat a cupcake – and enjoy it! Healthy living is just as much about your mental wellbeing as it is your physical. If you're obsessing over every carb and gram of fat, you're not leading a life that's as fulfilled as it can be. A healthy lifestyle is about so much more than calories in versus calories out. It's a balance of those things as well as your loving relationships, your career, and your spirituality. It's about nourishing your soul as much as your body. In short, you should NEVER deprive yourself of something you want. Life is simply too short. Remember that wherever you are in your life and your wellness journey, you didn't get there overnight.

Similarly, wherever it is you would *like* to be, you won't get to overnight either. Have patience, make small changes, and revel in your success when you start seeing results. Remember this is about being HEALTHY, not skinny (that's right, I said it). Healthy equals happy. Skinny? Not always.

Working Girl's Exercise

In a typical day, what do you eat? Do you find you consume a lot of processed foods, and not too many whole foods? Do you pay more attention to the calorie count of what you're eating than the ingredients?

_____

_____

_____

What are two or three healthy whole foods you will add in to your day? (Ex. "I will add a serving of broccoli to my dinner plate" or "I will add a side of vegetable soup to my lunch".)

_____

_____

_____

CHAPTER 10

Keeping Work at Work

"You can't do a good job, if your job is all you do."

— UNKNOWN

MANY OF US have professions which require us to take our work home with us. Even more of us take enough emotion home from work with us that it *seems* like we're taking our work home.

Think about this (and try not to feel depressed). We spend, at a minimum, eight and a half hours a day in the office, including lunch (which by now you are consistently breaking for). If we're lucky, our commute is less than thirty minutes a day but in most cases will be upwards of two hours round trip. We take an hour to prepare for work in the morning, and at least an hour at night when you factor in preparing lunches and laying out clothes. That's more than half of the day! Still want to take your work home with you?

Let's talk boundaries. First, clear your mind. Think of one or two challenges you face when it comes to leaving your work at the door (use the "Exercise" page at the end of this chapter to take notes). Does your boss call you at night? Does the nature of your job require after-hours attention like lesson planning or case work? Or do you just find yourself thinking about work when you're with your family?

Whatever the obstacle, decide on a strategy to handle it and stick to your guns. Politely tell your boss that you need time to relax and reset at night in order to continue to do your best work during the day. Same goes for coworkers, if someone in your office loves to call you at night to discuss the daily drama.

Implement strict home office hours. This applies to both the hours you spend working at home and the amount of time you spend talking about it. Make a rule with your spouse that you each get five minutes to talk about your day, and then move on. Designate a "Power Hour" – for example, between the hours of 7:00 and 8:00 you focus on your work with no disruptions, and the rest of the evening is work-free.

Establish a "No Phone Zone". A great idea is to ban cell phones from the dinner table, so that everyone has a chance to focus on each other. Another idea is to shut your phone off one hour before lights out and give your mind a chance to wind down.

Maintain as much (mental) distance as possible in your off hours. Even though you can't hop a plane every Friday afternoon and head to a tropical island, you can certainly do it in your head. When you're away from the office, be away mind, body and soul. Focus on the things that make you whole. Once you get used to distancing yourself from your work, you'll find you can do it even on your lunch break. Any chance you get to step away, clear your mind, and take some deep breaths - even if it's only for a few minutes - is incredibly restorative. In time those boundaries will become completely natural.

It takes time to establish these distinctions between your work life and your home life. Often times, it takes a certain wakeup call to cause you to realize that you are lacking proper boundaries. For me, it was realizing that I always came home looking tired and defeated, prompting my family to ask me "Bad day?" over and over. I knew it must not be any fun to have a miserable person coming through the door every afternoon, and I started to learn to leave work at work.

Working Girl's Exercise

What are one or two obstacles you face when it comes to leaving your work at the door?

_____

_____

_____

What will you do differently? (Ex. "I will implement a 'No Phone Zone' at the dinner table" or "I will turn off all technologies one hour before bedtime".)

_____

_____

_____

CHAPTER 11

Finding Your Happy/ Healthy Work Balance

"Never get so busy making a living that you forget to make a life."

— Unknown

I'VE HAD A strong work ethic all my life. I do my work imme-diately and efficiently. I keep my promises. I show up on time and stay until the job is done. I follow up, I'm con-sistent. I've always felt guilty about taking sick days. I am widely recognized as a diligent, hard worker and am well respected by people I've worked with.

I do not, however, work late nights and weekends. I don't take my work home with me. I don't dwell on things that happened at the office when I'm not there (or much when I am there). I know when the work day begins and when it ends. I maintain balance and consider "work" and "not at work" to be two completely separate lives. One does not interfere with the other.

There are four aspects of a balanced lifestyle, aside from the food on your plate: being physically active, nourishing loving relationships, practicing some sort of spirituality, and having a satisfying career.

For a long time, I attributed my "perfect balance" to hav-ing an extremely fulfilling home life that overcompen-sated for my not-so-satisfying work life. Whenever I found myself upset or stressed out during the 9-to-5, I simply checked in at home, whether it be by physically calling a member of my family or mentally recalling a memory or person I cherished. This worked until I unexpectedly lost my dad, and suddenly my personal life was shattered right along with my heart. Working became unbearable, and it wasn't long before I realized I needed to make a change. Since I couldn't change my personal situation, I had to do something about work.

Just to be clear, when I say "do something about work", I don't mean anger-quit, walk out, or even normal-quit. Sometimes, finding peace at work – or in any aspect of life – is as simple as shifting your mindset. And I really do mean, SIMPLE. It might not seem that way at first, but once you accept the fact that no one controls your thoughts, your emotions, and your reactions other than YOU, it becomes second nature.

So how do you achieve this "mindset shift"? You guessed it – I have tips! Let's dive in…

Have something on the calendar to look forward to. … Because sometimes, all it takes is a reminder that there's life on the outside. A week or so before the start of a new month I'll take a look at my calendar and see what holidays, birthdays and other events are coming up and get planning! My whole life people have told me "Just wait until you get older, you won't care about things like celebrating birthdays anymore". All I could think was, "Wow, I really hope that's not true". Why aren't we celebrating birthdays and holidays anymore? Because we're too busy at work?! How sad! Make the decision now to make friends and family more of a priority. Try to plan something at least every other week, more often if your schedule permits it. Having an active social life is an incredibly effective stress management technique and will have you feeling infinitely better at the office. Bonus points if you can make plans with a friend who never ceases to crack you up!

Determine your happy place, and go there often. Inner peace is achieved in different ways by different people. Close your eyes and go to your happy place. Where are you? On a beach? Out on a run? Out to dinner with your friends? In a yoga class? When you're all settled in to your happy place, take a few deep breaths and center yourself.

Find a creative outlet. Get a hobby! Try journaling, create a vision board, or make a scrapbook. You can even channel your creative energy into a few new recipes! If you're at a loss for ideas (and you have a few hours to spare) try Pinterest for inspiration. Zen coloring books are a wonderfully therapeutic way to unwind, and how great is it that we finally have a grown-up excuse to use crayons? In all seriousness, finding a creative outlet that works for you is an excellent stress management tool.

Stay active, no matter how busy you are. If I'm having a particularly busy week and I can't go out for a run, I feel the difference in a very real way. I'm just not myself, I'm irritable, and I feel physically heavy. Once you get into a routine with progressively increasing your daily movement, you'll see what I mean. Observe the difference in how you feel on weeks you are very active, versus weeks you aren't. Exercising regularly has been proven to lower stress levels time and time again! In Chapter Five I shared a few suggestions with you for incorporating movement into your day even when you can't carve out an hour for the gym. Refer back to them when you feel like you need a little extra activity in a particularly busy work week.

Working Girl's Exercise

How balanced do you feel between home and work? Which one outweighs the other, from a stress standpoint?

_____

_____

_____

What can you do to alleviate some of the stress and achieve a better personal/professional balance? (Ex. "I will plan a girls' day with my friends" or "I will finally break out those vacation photos from last year and make a scrapbook".)

_____

_____

_____

CHAPTER 12

Avoid the Mid-Afternoon Slump

THE MID-AFTERNOON SLUMP. You know what I'm talking about. You conquered the morning rush. You got through lunch. And yet somehow… it's STILL not 5:00. Grogginess sets in. You start dragging your feet. Your mind feels cloudy. And each minute feels longer than the one before it.

Yuck! What a terrible way to feel at any time, but especially every day! Afternoon is basically the best part of the day – it's the only time of day that the sun is out no matter what time of year it is, the day is at its warmest and the energy is at its best. Forget the slump, we've got work to do! I don't know about you all, but during the winter months when we have those infamously shorter days, I find myself (despite my best efforts) pretty low on energy by the time evening rolls around. That's why I strive to be as productive as possible during the afternoon. I find that my energy is boundless and I feel more positive - there is simply more pep in my step. If I found myself longing for a nap every day at 3pm, nothing would get done.

Here are a few ways to beat the afternoon blues…

Beware of the lunchtime "food coma". Have you ever ordered takeout with your coworkers and felt like falling asleep immediately after lunch? It's because your body is now using so much energy to digest the heavy meal that it can't keep up with its other processes as efficiently. In

Chapter Nine we broke down the basics of a balanced plate – half vegetables, a quarter healthy whole grains, and a quarter clean protein. Stick to those guidelines even when ordering out, and be careful not to overeat. Restaurants usually give you way more than one portion size so split it in half and save some for tomorrow's lunch. If you have time, take a short walk or sip some warm lemon water after you eat. I've found that doing either of these things help me to digest a big meal. Also, if you ARE eating a salt-heavy meal, as most takeout tends to be, make sure you're following it up with plenty of water.

Skip the coffee; try fruit instead. I'm speaking from personal experience here, I've never actually read anything saying that fruit has the same effect on your energy level as coffee – and, a coffee lover to the core, this trick only works for me in the afternoon. If you tried to give me strawberries in place of my AM jolt, I probably wouldn't be too happy with you! But at 3 or 4 in the afternoon, when I need a little pick-me-up and I'm in between meals, I've found that a plate of fruit is super refreshing and gives me the boost I need at that time of day.

Take a walk. You should be doing this regularly throughout the day anyway, but when you're feeling that mid-day drowsiness kicking in, take a short walk. Do a lap of the office or go outside for fresh air if you can. Take a few conscious breaths, clear your head, and recharge briefly before you head back to your desk.

Know your power songs. No matter what I'm doing, it's made ten times better when I can stop for a dance break. Of course, jumping up for a dance at your desk might earn you a couple of confused glances from your coworkers (or worse!), but you can pop in an earbud for a minute and listen to that song that always lifts you up. If your office setting permits it, keep a radio at your desk. Listening to music all day long may be a little distracting for you and your coworkers alike, but it can be handy when you need a quick boost.

Working Girl's Exercise

Do you suffer from the dreaded mid-afternoon slump? What do you find is typically the cause – a heavy lunch, lack of sleep the night before, not enough breaks during the day? Something else? Identifying the problem will make it easier to correct!

_____

_____

_____

Now that you know what's weighing you down, what are a few actions steps you can take to help you thrive at 3pm?

_____

_____

_____

CHAPTER 13

How to Pass the Test of Patience with Flying Colors

In Chapter Eleven I talked a lot about my work/life balance. I said that my idea of "balance" was overcompensating for my unhappiness in the work place with an abundance of happiness in my personal life (not a bad solution to a state of imbalance, right? Too much happiness at home?). Once I lost my dad, however, and my situation at home changed completely I no longer felt at peace in ANY aspect of my life. Something needed to change.

On my path to making this change – heading to nutrition school to learn about holistic health and wellness, publishing my books, raising my voice about heart disease – I learned a lot about myself and the way I viewed "balance" in the past. It's as finite as mathematics: having more of one thing to make up for a lack of something else is essentially the definition of UNBALANCED.

One important thing I've learned, which I've mentioned several times throughout this book and I wholeheartedly believe now that I've experienced it, is that if you can't change your situation, you must change your relationship to it.

So what exactly does that mean? You can't simply flip a switch and change your feelings, right? (Though wouldn't that be nice?)

While there is no magic on/off switch, the truth is that changing your relationship to your job CAN be very easy. The choice to embrace your situation is a conscious one that you have the power to make on a daily basis. As you learn to tune into what your body is telling you and figure out what makes you feel balanced and centered (which we will dig deeper into in a moment), making the conscious choice to accept – even enjoy! – your work will seem like second nature.

Determine what points during the day you feel stressed. Is it first thing in the morning when you see twenty new emails in your inbox? Around noon, when you feel like you've put in a full day but you're only halfway there? Or does the overwhelm hit at the end of the day, when it's time to go home but your desk is still piled high with files? Observe how you feel throughout the day and recognize when the stress starts to kick in. Next time it happens, don't just ignore it. Do something about it. Stop what you're doing and take a few deep breaths. Take a walk, take a music break, or chat with a coworker for a few minutes. Close your eyes and go to the happy place we unearthed in Chapter Eleven. Do these mini-resets as many times as you need to throughout the day.

Eat regularly. This may seem like strange advice, but I've been there many times: Something that shouldn't bother me much has me totally fired up for an unexplained reason. I hear myself, I know I'm overreacting, yet it's hard to calm down. You've seen the commercials on TV - not that you needed to. You KNOW that hungry equals cranky. In the hustle and bustle of office life, it's easy to forget that you haven't eaten in hours. Keep a stash of healthy snacks in your desk drawer, something simple like almonds or trail mix (refer to Chapter Four: The Art of Healthy Snacking), for a quick fix. Before you overreact or lose your patience in a situation, ask yourself if you're simply hungry.

Act, don't react. Think before you speak. If you need time to collect your thoughts, tell the person on the receiving end that you will get back to them as soon as possible. If you're particularly short on patience, communicate via email so you have time to phrase what you want to say in a professional and appropriate manner.

Patience is a virtue... but it sure can be hard to come by sometimes. Once you learn what triggers your stress and figure out what helps you keep your sanity, you'll find it takes a lot more for you to lose your cool than it once did.

Working Girl's Exercise

Be honest: One a scale from one to ten, how patient are you? Observing your stress level throughout the day, list your triggers. Determining what sets you off will make it easier to determine how to calm down.

_____

_____

_____

What will you do to keep these triggers from getting the best of you? (Ex. "I will close my eyes and count to ten the next time I'm feeling stressed" or "I will take a walk around the office before I respond to a coworker who is getting on my nerves".)

_____

_____

_____

CHAPTER 14

Not-So-Happy Hour

It NEVER FAILED. At every single work luncheon I have ever attended, a conversation about my eating habits ensued. A typical in-office work party usually consisted of one or a combination of the following: bagels, heroes stuffed with meat and cheese, pizza, chips and soda. I, a clean-eating vegetarian, tried to either make my plate look full with food I COULD eat, if I could find any, got food for my coworker and gave it to her quietly later on, or if I could I skipped the party altogether.

I was always met with a flurry of questions – "Why aren't you eating?" "Are you on a diet?" "You're a vegetarian? Why? Since when?" "Well there's no meat on the pizza, why can't you eat the pizza?"

I absolutely implore you; don't ever put someone in the awkward position of having to explain their dietary habits to you. To each his own, okay? Curiosity is fine but check the judgment at the door. This constant line of questioning really made me come to dread social functions at work. I couldn't understand why we always had to be rewarded in sugary, processed foods. Don't get me wrong – the gesture of gratitude from upper management was appreciated, but almost always resulted in me feeling uncomfortable and having to defend my lifestyle. No fun.

Years of politely declining a piece of the six-foot hoagie has taught me a few tricks on taking the healthy road during office parties, happy hours, and other social engagements, that I'm happy to pass along to you now.

Eat before you go. Fill up on your brought-from-home lunch before heading to the party/luncheon/happy hour. Allow yourself a treat when you get there if you want, but eating before you go will curb any temptation to devour the pizza and sandwiches. Better yet, bring a healthy dish to contribute to the festivities! Show your coworkers how delicious healthy eating can be, and set a good example for them.

Stick to a one-drink limit. Too much alcohol can quickly turn an after-work gathering into a not-so-happy hour. Sip one glass of wine over the course of the night, or order a non-alcoholic but sparkly beverage. Be sure to alternate with water to help you stay at the top of your game and avoid any awkward encounters with your coworkers – or worse, your boss.

Stick with the veggie platter or the salads. Load up on the leafy greens and enjoy your work luncheon without any questions from your coworkers! (Well, with fewer questions.) A good rule of thumb when trying to eat clean under difficult circumstances (i.e. a party) is to fill up on veggies first, and then indulge as you wish. This way your body has a chance to absorb the nutrients it needs, and by the time you're done you won't crave the sugary, processed foods as much anyway.

Have your "elevator speech" ready. This is your perfunctory answer when those inevitable questions arise. And try not to get offended when people ask. Chances are they're not judging, just curious. Perhaps they see you eating healthy and are interested in doing the same.

Don't be too hard on yourself. If you find you ate one too many cookies at the holiday party, don't beat yourself up. And by all means, don't use it as an excuse to continue eating bad because you think the whole day is a lost cause. Drink some warm water with lemon (or plain old water will do the trick in a pinch), take a walk if you can or at least do a lap of the office, and shake it off (or if it's that kind of party, dance if off!).

Working Girl's Exercise

Let's break it down: What's the vibe at your office parties? Are you trying to eat healthy while everyone else is gorging on chips? Do you feel like a bit of an outcast? Do you find yourself overindulging out of temptation?

_____

_____

_____

List a few action steps you're going to take to ensure you stay true to your happy healthy self in all social situations where food is involved. Will you eat before you go? Alternate alcoholic drinks with water? Contribute a healthy dish to the party?

_____

_____

_____

CHAPTER 15

Live and Let Go

"Forgiveness is a gift you give yourself."

— TONY ROBBINS

ONE OF THE hardest things I've had to do in my professional life was learn to forgive the people who have wronged me and moved on. As we talked about early on in Chapter Three, office settings are unnatural. They force people together for the majority of their respective waking hours – people who most likely haven't chosen to be placed together. It's impossible for every person to be a perfect match for every person they sit near. Even the most easygoing people are bound to bump heads once in a while when they're together all day, every day. Emotions can run high in stressful corporate environments (and most other working environments, I'm sure), where staffers are typically overworked, underpaid, and facing deadlines.

When the going gets rough, remember that this too shall pass. I don't typically advise people to "look forward to" anything, in the sense of looking ahead to Friday the moment your shift starts on Monday or counting the days until vacation starting January first. Have you ever seen the movie "Click"? Adam Sandler's character is given a remote control that allows him to fast forward through unpleasant events in his life, like arguments and boring meetings, but he loses control and essentially fast-forwards through his whole life. I really encourage you to stay focused on and find the good in the present moment – and if you can't find anything, create something. Call a friend and schedule an outing. Plan something special for an upcoming birthday in the family. That being said, some days are rougher than others and in those moments, rest assured that 5:00 will be here soon.

Working Girl's Exercise

What are you holding on to that you're ready to let go of?

_____

_____

_____

Now – LET IT GO. List two or three mantras or reminders to give yourself every time you feel that unnecessary frustration creeping up on you.

_____

_____

_____

CHAPTER 16

Know When it's Time to Move On

"It's time to move on, time to get goin'
What lies ahead I have no way of knowin'
But under my feet baby, grass is growin'"

— TOM PETTY, *TIME TO MOVE ON*

THE AVERAGE FULL-TIME employee spends two thousand hours or more a year at work. Over the course of forty years, that's eighty thousand hours or more than nine years of your life. That's an awful lot of time to spend in a job that makes you genuinely unhappy.

I realize how hard it can be to imagine your dream job. Life is long, and it's almost impossible to say what kind of career you will want thirty years down the road (or even five years). If you're not sure if you're in the right position for you, ask yourself these questions:

It's Sunday night. How are you feeling?

- A. Fine. After all, it's the weekend!
- B. Okay, but bummed hat the weekend is almost over.
- C. Complete and utter dread.

At work, are you:

- A. Giving it your all. You never know when an opportunity for a promotion might come up!
- B. Not thrilled to be there, but you make the best of it.
- C. Clock-watching. Is it 5 yet? ...How about now?

How much appreciation are you getting for the job you're doing?

    A. I know my boss is grateful for my hard work. He/she tells me all the time.

    B. Some, my boss doesn't seek me out often but my annual reviews are always decent.

    C. My boss doesn't know I'm alive/is constantly demeaning me.

If you answered mostly A's… You have a great gig, and that's awesome! Not many people can say that they truly enjoy going to work. Just make sure you're not giving up too much of yourself to please your boss – remember, it's all about that work/life balance. If you can honestly say you've got the best of both worlds, you're in great shape!

If you answered mostly B's… You probably have a good relationship with your job. You give it your best shot (most of the time, anyway) but you know where to draw the line between your work life and home life. Plan a little happy hour on Wednesday with your girlfriends to keep your spirits up, and you're good to go.

If you answered mostly C's… Ask yourself why. What exactly is it about your job that's bringing you down? Your boss?

Your duties? The hours? Benefits? Write it down and be specific. Is there anything you can do to change it? I've gone to my boss MANY times over the years to express concerns about various aspects of my job. Because she always knew I was coming from a place of sincerity, and she knows I do my best each and every day, she always listened and tried to work with me. I realize not everyone is that lucky, but it doesn't hurt to try. Otherwise, evaluate your other options. See if you're in line for a promotion or if there is an opening in another department you can check out. Ask if there are different tasks you can take on to mix up your routine a little. If you're feeling that badly, you may need a chance of pace altogether. It never hurts to look around a little, maybe send out your resume to that company you've been dying to work for!

Let me be clear: I am in NO WAY encouraging you to march into your boss's office tomorrow and hand in your resignation letter. Likewise, I'm not telling you to settle into a job that may make you happy on a superficial level if deep down, something else calls to you. All I'm trying to do here is give you some perspective. Know that you are not a prisoner to your current situation. If you're not in a place right now where you can or want to change your job, you can ALWAYS change your relationship to it.

What do I mean by that? As I touched on in Chapter Fifteen, I went through a period where for no good reason (but every good reason, I thought at the time), I was angry all the time. I mean, absolutely seething. I didn't want to talk to anyone, I was fired up every day, and I cried all the time. It's well worth it to mention that I've since cut most sugar out of my diet, and I'd encourage you to start making steps to do the same. Once I realized that sugar was responsible for my sudden mood swings, my life changed. There IS a relationship between your food and your mood – a significant one. What you eat affects how you feel and how you act. As you take steps to improve your health, try food journaling (tracking what you're eating, when you're eating it, how much water you're drinking, and how you feel before and after). Notice how eating more healthy whole foods and fewer sugary, processed foods improves your stress level and your overall outlook.

M&M's aside, I finally realized that the unnecessary anger I was harboring was only hurting myself. It wasn't getting me anywhere and it certainly wasn't improving my situation. I made a conscious decision to change my attitude. I made the same conscious decision the next day, and the day after that. Eventually, it became a habit. Before long, this conscious mindfulness - combined with walking on my lunch breaks, eating cleaner, finding reasons to laugh more, and leading a fulfilling "non-work" life - caused my entire mindset to shift. I felt more centered every day. I found peace where before there was only chaos. I had changed my relationship with work. Monday? Bring it on. Friday? That's cool too.

Working Girl's Exercise

How do you handle your current job situation on a mental/emotional level? How do you WISH you handled it?

_____

_____

_____

List three POSITIVE aspects of your job. Refer back to them whenever you need a boost.

_____

_____

_____

CONCLUSION

This Life is All You Get – Don't Live it For Your Company

"Your work is going to fill a large part of your life, and the only way to be truly satisfied is to do what you believe is great work. And the only way to do great work is to love what you do. If you haven't found it yet, keep looking. Don't settle. As with all matters of the heart, you'll know it when you find it."

— STEVE JOBS

PEOPLE AREN'T ALWAYS quick to empathize with each other, but the truth of the matter is that regardless of what we have going on at home, having a full time job is absolutely exhausting. You're gone for most of the day, away from your home and your family, and you spend a lot of the time you *are* home preparing just to go back to work. The world would be a much better place if everyone tried a little harder to remember that we're *all* struggling sometimes, and loved each other a little bit more.

No matter what your job situation is or what steps you can/ are willing to take to make it better, remember this: this one life is all you get. There are no do-overs. Each moment is fleeting, and then it's gone forever. Don't be the person who looks back in ten, twenty, or fifty years wondering where the time went, only to realize it was spent at work, preparing for work, or thinking about work. Spend time with your family. Spend time with yourself. Learn the things that make you happy, and do them often. Cherish and make the most of your "off" hours so you can feel more fulfilled during your "on" hours. Remember that no matter what happens during your workday, it is only your workday. The important memories are waiting to be made at home. Do your best and show respect to everyone who crosses your path, but check your work at the office door. Once you implement some of these tools and strike a balance between home and work, you will find yourself in an upmost state of peace in both settings. You won't need one to counteract the other. You CAN have the best of both worlds.

You are now equipped with all of the secrets of a happy healthy working girl. Now go out there and become one!

About the Author

KIMBERLY PETROSINO IS a Holistic Health Coach who previously authored "The Small Change Solution: A 52 Step Guide to Getting the Naturally Healthy Lifestyle You Want". When she lost her father to a sudden heart attack, she made it her mission to spread awareness about the importance of healthy living to as many people as she can reach. In her spare time, Kimberly loves running, scrapbooking, experimenting in the kitchen, and being with people who inspire her and keep her centered. She is committed to helping others stay stress-free, happy, and heart healthy. Find out more at www.happyhealthyhearts.net or on Twitter @hh_hearts.

Interested in having Kimberly speak at your school, office, or other event? Visit www.happyhealthyhearts.net and click "Connect" or send an email to kimberly@happyhealthyhearts.net.

Final Thoughts + Acknowledgments

THIS BOOK WAS a long time in the making. When I started writing it, I was living one life. By the time I finished. I was living entirely another. Some who were once key players in my inner circle, I'm no longer in communication with. I drew inspiration from unlikely sources – A woman who I've only known a few short years, but empowers me in ways she'll probably never understand (even though I tell her as often as I get the chance!) and gives me a role model to aspire to. New friends who turned out to be the accountability partners I needed in the moment, encouraging me to keep writing. A fabulous group of *shining* women who make up my most solid support system and inspire me each with their own uniqueness and ability to push through their fears and boundaries every single day. Colleagues who went above and beyond in ways I'm undeserving of – to lend an ear, a shoulder to cry on, a surface to bounce off of, and to give me a space to open up without judgment, unconditionally and every day. Clients who move me on a daily basis with their boundless energy and determination to change what doesn't work and achieve their goals. When this book was nothing more than a figment of my imagination and notes scribbled on whatever scrap of paper was laying around the moment I had a brainstorm, I thought my nearest and dearest would remain so for the rest of my life (that's right, "friends forever" is not just for the high school-aged!). I was POSITIVE that my plan would unfold to my exact specifications, because I believed in it so strongly. Well the universe had something else in mind for me, and here I am now with another book that turned into something totally different from what I'd originally dreamed up, living a life totally different from what I'd originally dreamed up.

And you know what? I wouldn't change a moment of it.

With that being said…

To my sisters in the New Self Health Movement – You changed my life in one weekend, each and every one of you, in your uniquely individual ways. You, my soul sisters, gave me the strength I needed to handle everything that came afterward. You pushed me outside the boundaries of my comfort zone into a life I thought existed only in the depths of my imagination. You taught me what it meant to love unconditionally, to share, to embrace, and to let go. You taught me that I could walk into a room in California on a beautiful October day, a bundle of nerves with no idea what to expect, and walk out three days later with a new family and renewed confidence in myself. I love you all so very much - you will never know the ways you impacted my life with your strength, your wisdom, and your true inner beauty.

To my coworkers through the years who inspired me to become a happier, healthier working girl – Changing jobs over the course of your life is always a growing experience but for me, never changing jobs proved even more so. It gives me a clean backdrop against which I can see all of the stages of my life – the people, the relationships, and the roller coaster of health and sickness and stress and peace. So many people I've had the pleasure of working with (and some, not so much) contributed to my journey. Coworkers I shared "healthy snacks" with; coworkers who tested my patience; coworkers who *taught* me patience. Some showed me the kind of person I want to be – others showed me the kind of person I *don't* want to be. I'm here now because of every one of you who touched my life, and I hope I've inspired some of you along the way as well. Thank you for being my friends, my sounding boards, my inspirations.

To my family – Thank you for your unfailing support of all of my endeavors and ideas, no matter how crazy they may seem. I'm grateful for your faith in me beyond words; especially during those times when I don't have faith in myself, it pushes me forward.

And last but never least, to my dad, who continues to inspire me, motivate me, and encourage me years after he was taken from me, all too soon – Thank you, thank you, thank you for this life, for being my reason to grow and build and help others, for being my inspiration for everything. EVERYTHING. As I tell you each and every single time I leave my pink lipstick marks all over your final resting place, I love you and miss you absolutely endlessly. Your life was taken unfairly and untimely and I promise I will never stop living mine with the upmost purpose and dedication to my vision, and to you, until the day I take my final breath.

www.ingramcontent.com/pod-product-compliance
Lightning Source LLC
Chambersburg PA
CBHW072205280526
45788CB00002B/880